I0790839

The Lively Adventures of Layla!

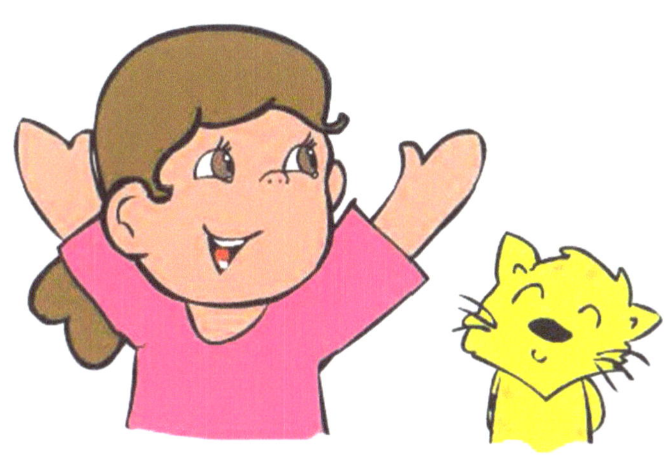

Written by Hiba Dahman Balfaqih

Illustrated by Jonathan Short

Dedicated to my giggly Layla!

"You're braver than you believe, and stronger than you seem, and smarter than you think." - Christopher Robin

I love you smelly feeta!

xx

H

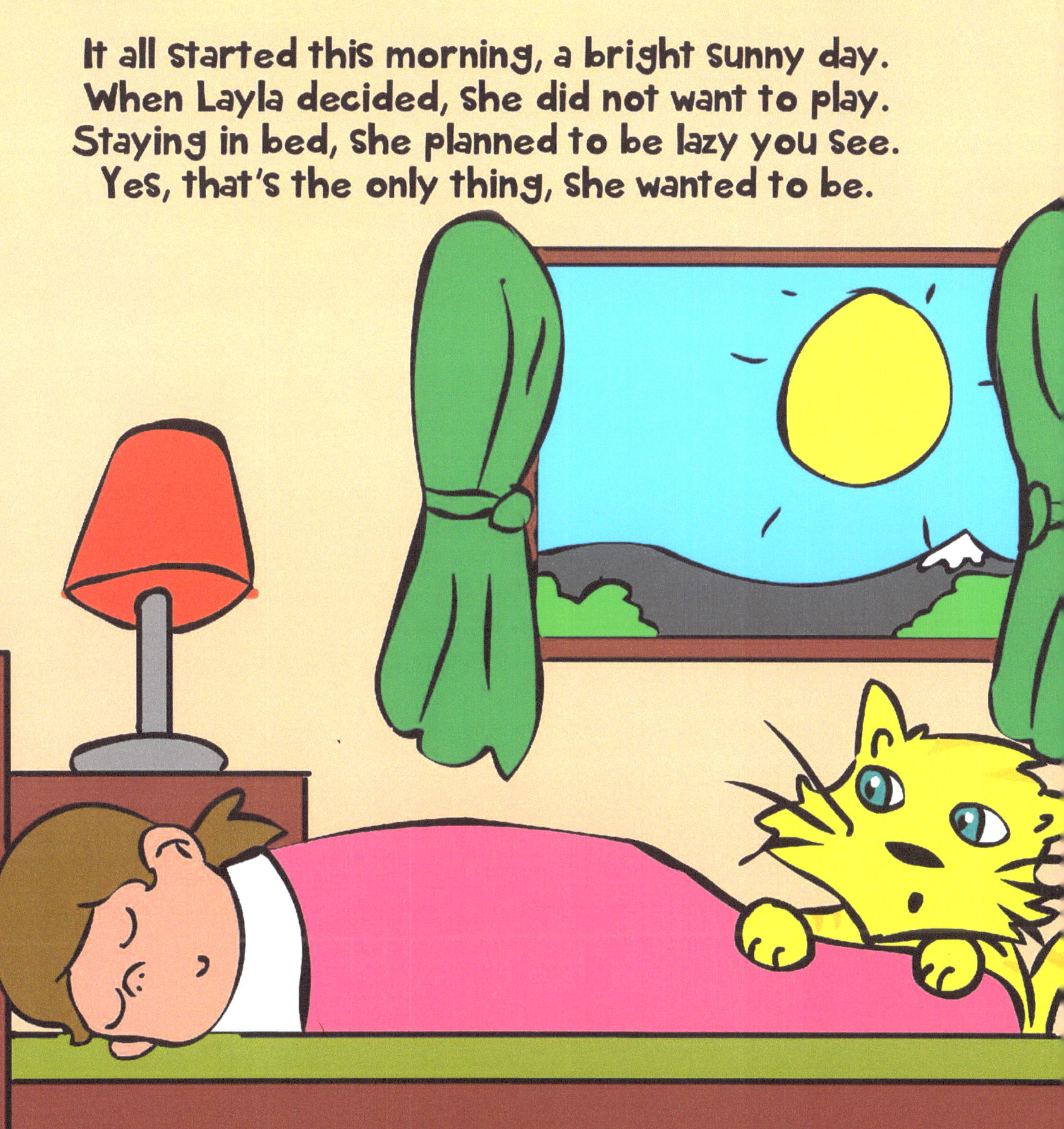

It all started this morning, a bright sunny day.
When Layla decided, she did not want to play.
Staying in bed, she planned to be lazy you see.
Yes, that's the only thing, she wanted to be.

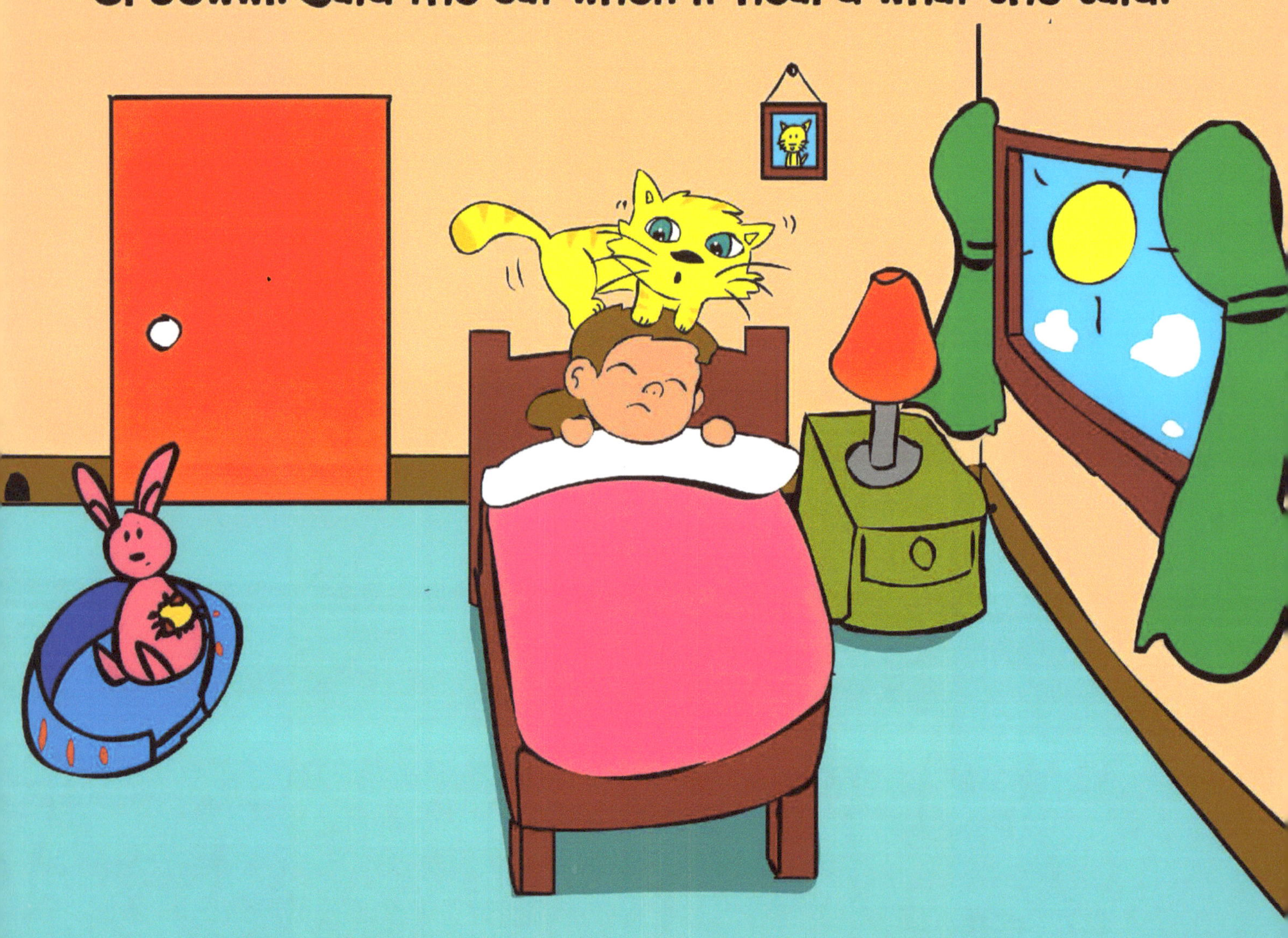

"Meow." Said her cat. Ollie was its name.
It jumped on her head, trying to play a game.
"No no. Not today, I am staying in bed."
Groowwl. Said the cat when it heard what she said.

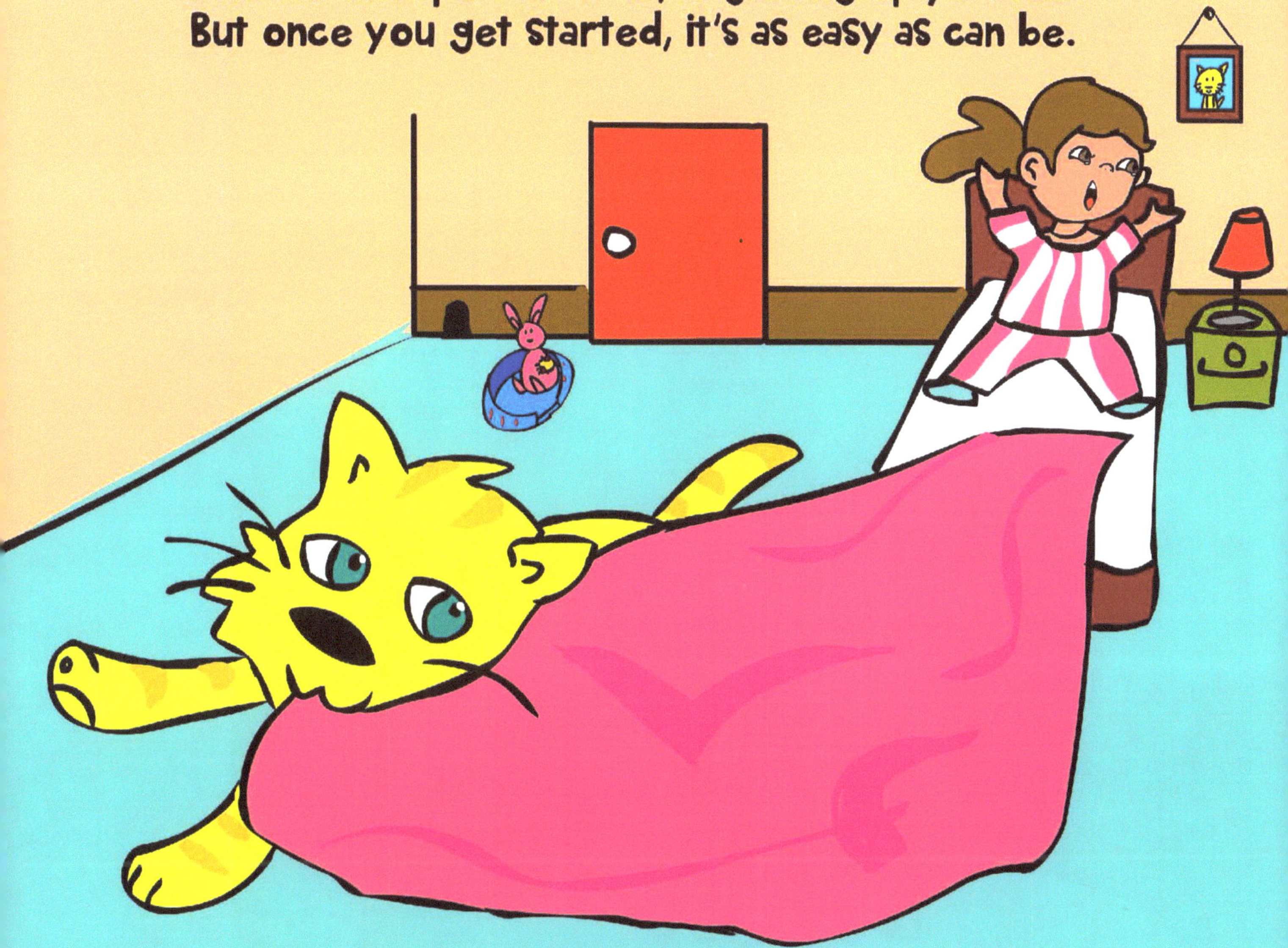

The cat pulled off the blankets, and dragged them around.
There were so many fun things that could always be found.
The hardest part of it all, is getting up you See.
But once you get started, it's as easy as can be.

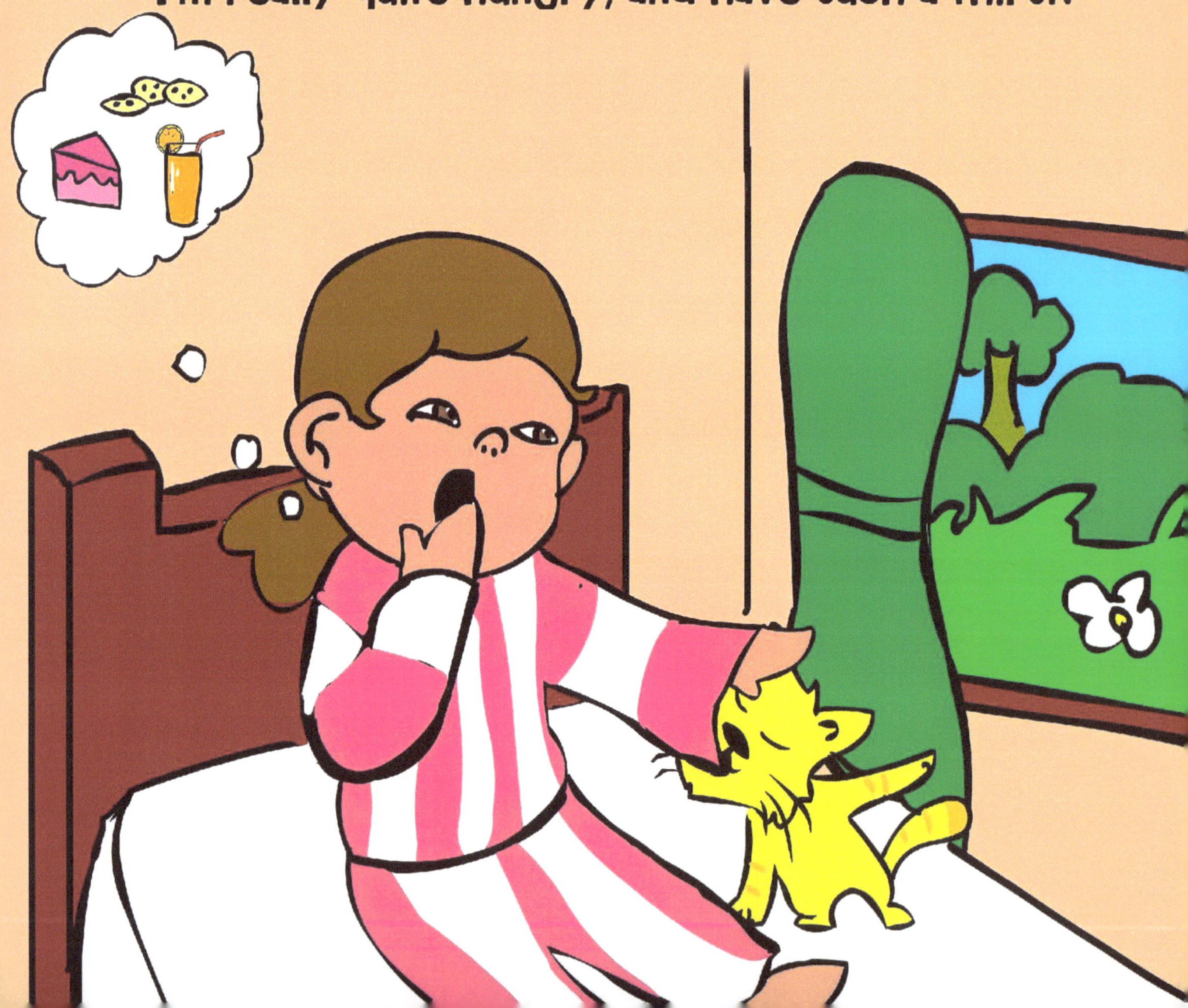

Layla stretched up her arms and let out a yawn.
Ollie pulled at her sleeve to play in the lawn.
"Not now." Layla said. I must eat something first.
"I'm really quite hungry, and have such a thirst."

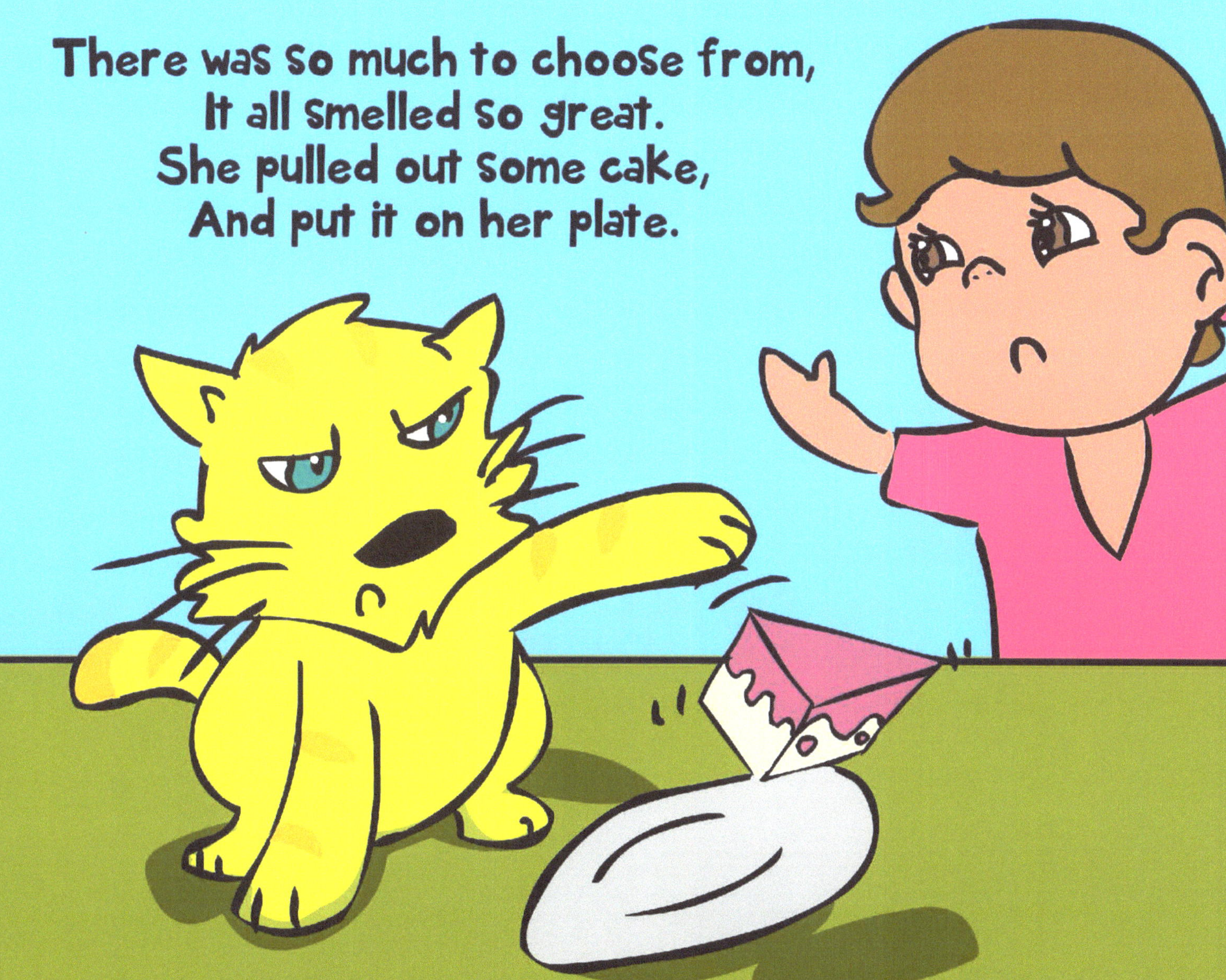
There was so much to choose from,
It all smelled so great.
She pulled out some cake,
And put it on her plate.

"HISS!" The cat knocked the cake
to the floor.
"Hey!" Layla shouted. "What did you do that for?"

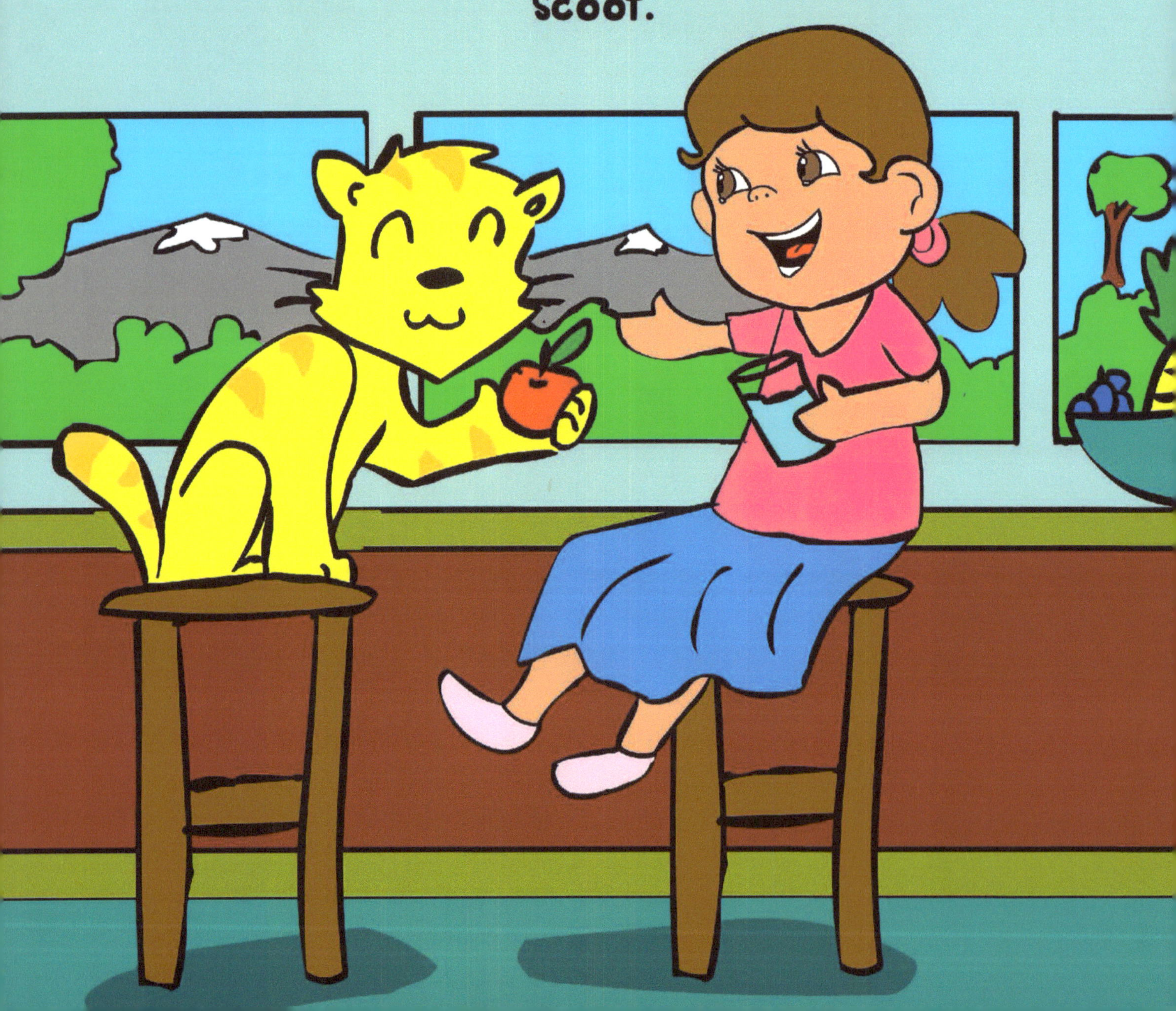

The cat jumped on the counter. She grabbed water and fruit.
Layla ate it all up, and jumped down with a scoot.

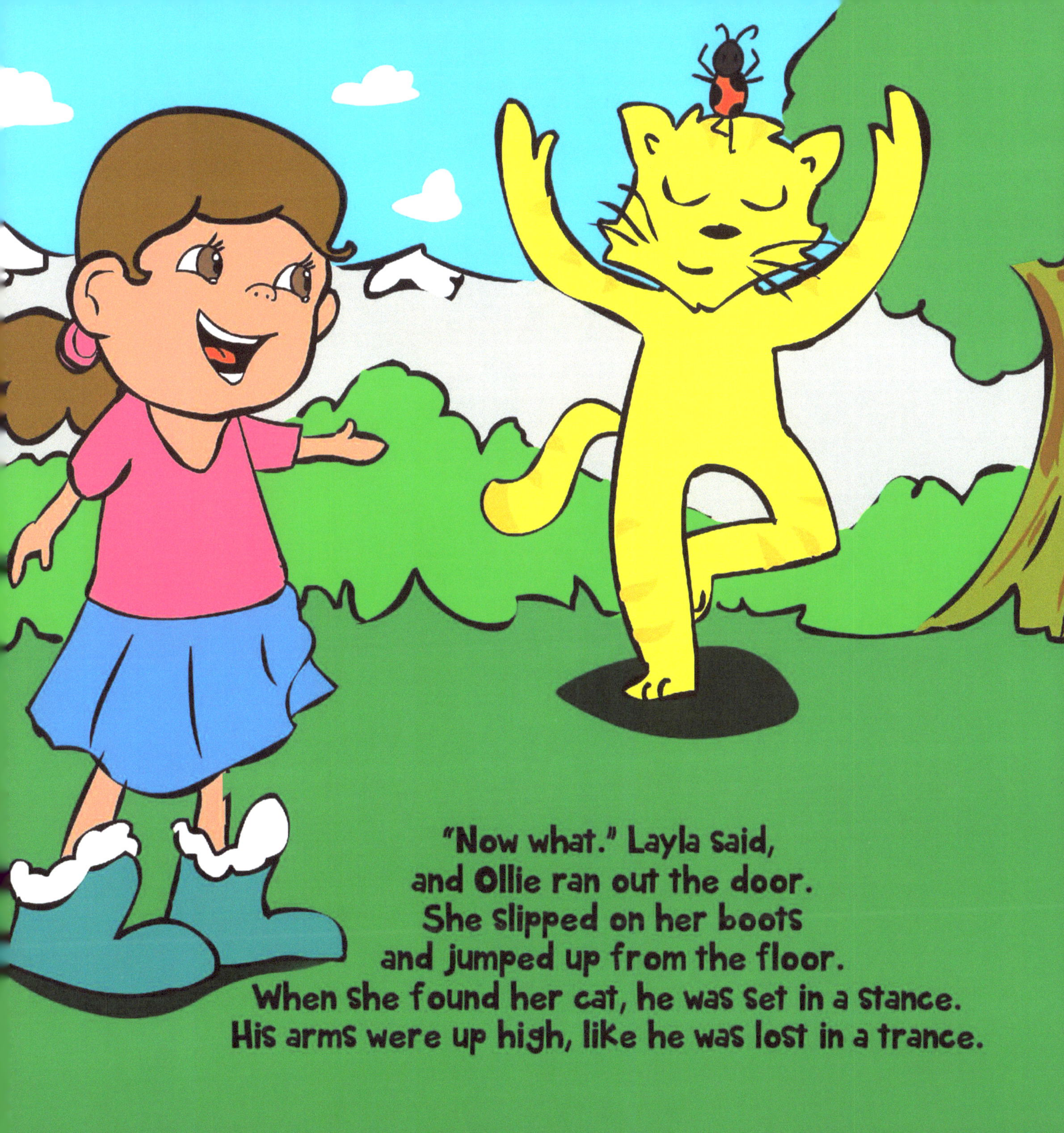

"Now what." Layla said,
and Ollie ran out the door.
She slipped on her boots
and jumped up from the floor.
When she found her cat, he was set in a stance.
His arms were up high, like he was lost in a trance.

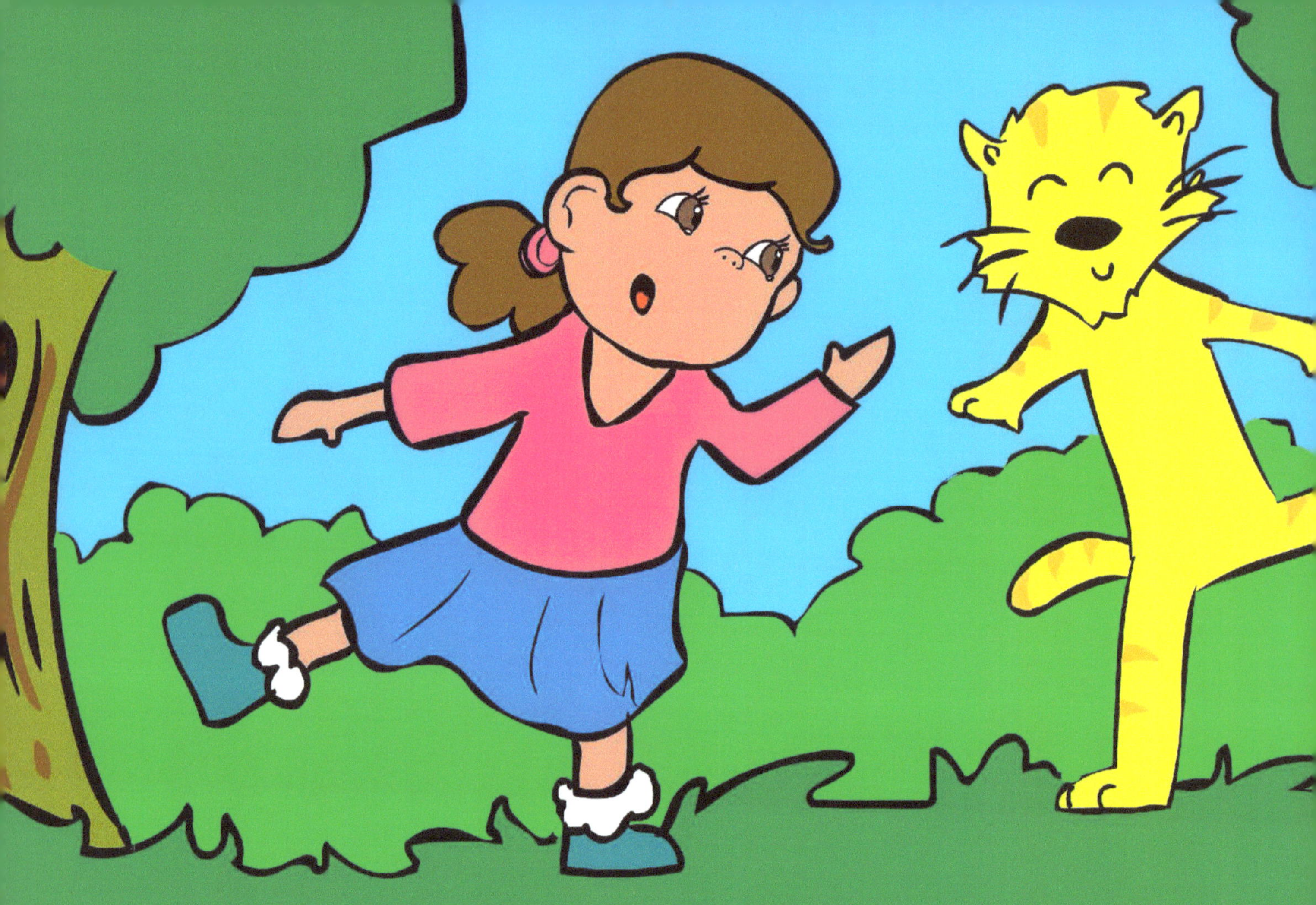

He was stretching up high, Layla did just the same.
So there it began, their fun stretching game.

First touch your toes, and count from one-to-ten.
Then take a small break, and do it over again.
Shake out your legs, the stretching is done.
Now it is time, to go play and run.

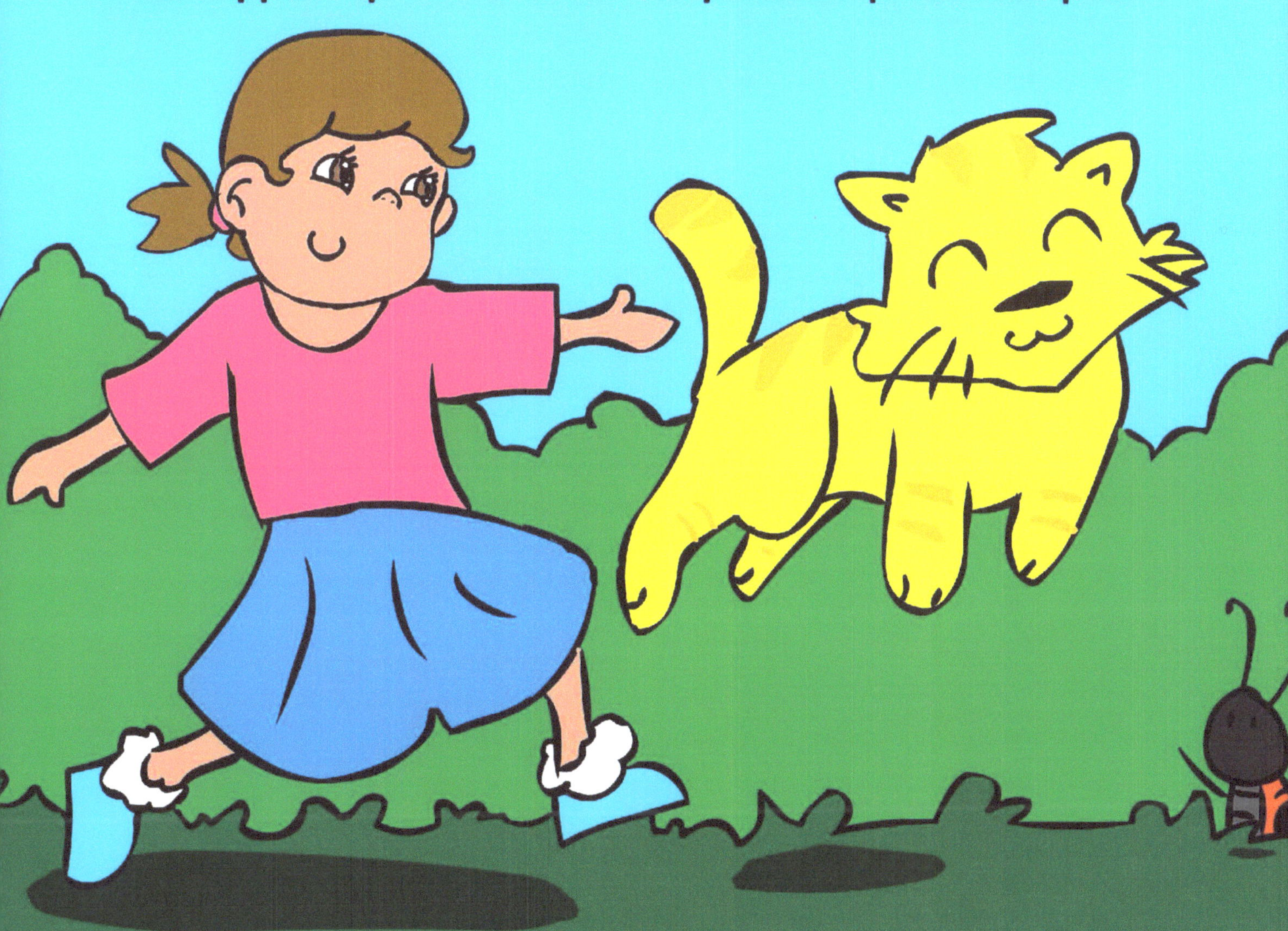

Layla and Ollie played for over an hour.
Eating fruit this morning, gave her so much power.
When they were all out of breath, they took a small pause.
Ollie lapped up some water he picked up with his paws.

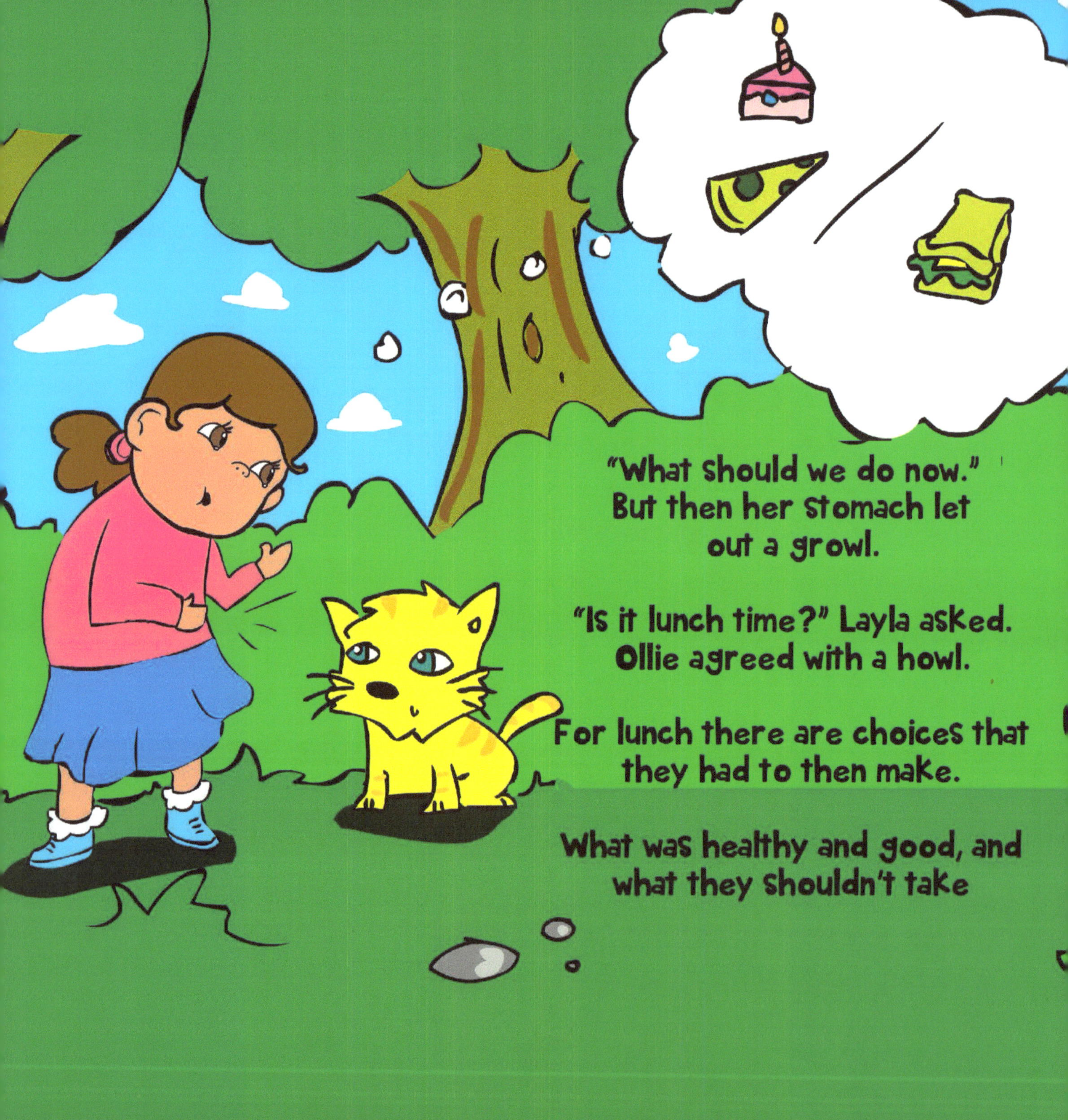

"What should we do now."
But then her stomach let
out a growl.

"Is it lunch time?" Layla asked.
Ollie agreed with a howl.

For lunch there are choices that
they had to then make.

What was healthy and good, and
what they shouldn't take

To make them really healthy, they can eat anything green.
Like salad or veggies, it is easier than it seems.
To make them really strong, they can eat meats or good beans.
It has protein and vitamins just like the greens.

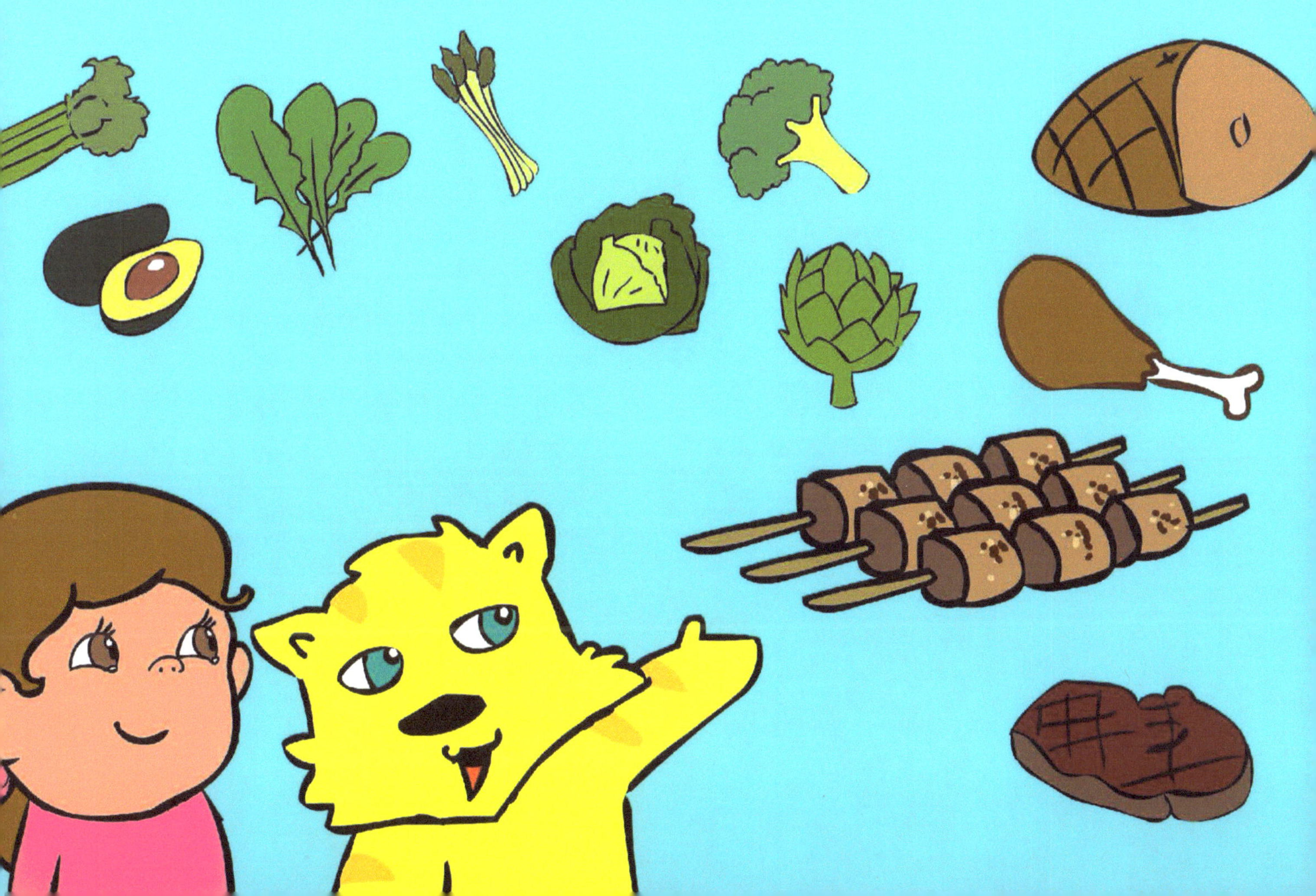

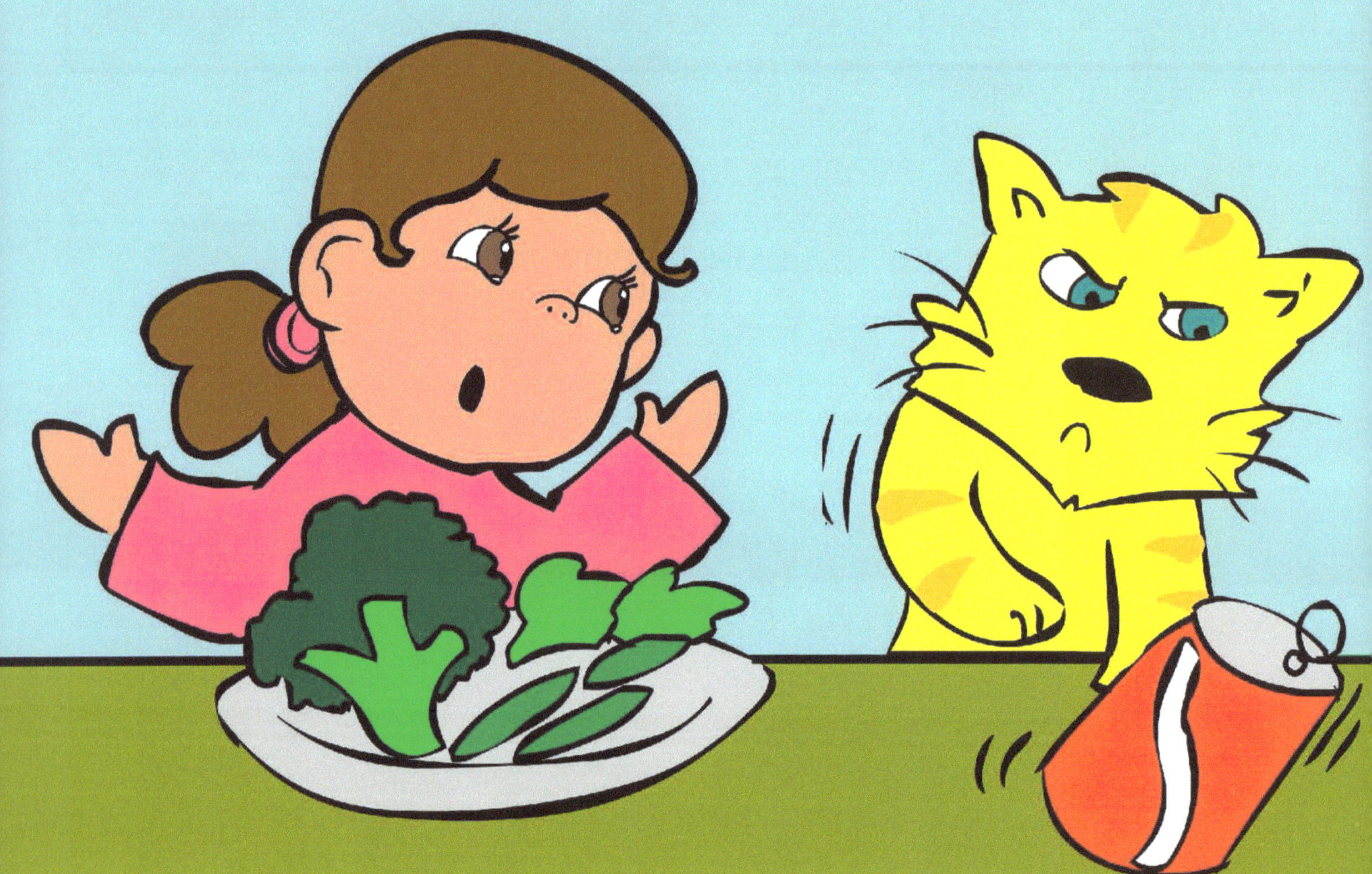

Layla reached for the soda, but Ollie slapped it away.
"Meow!" He said angrily, so she did not drink it that day.

She chose to drink water, it was delicious and cool.
Water hydrates the body, it's quite a useful tool.

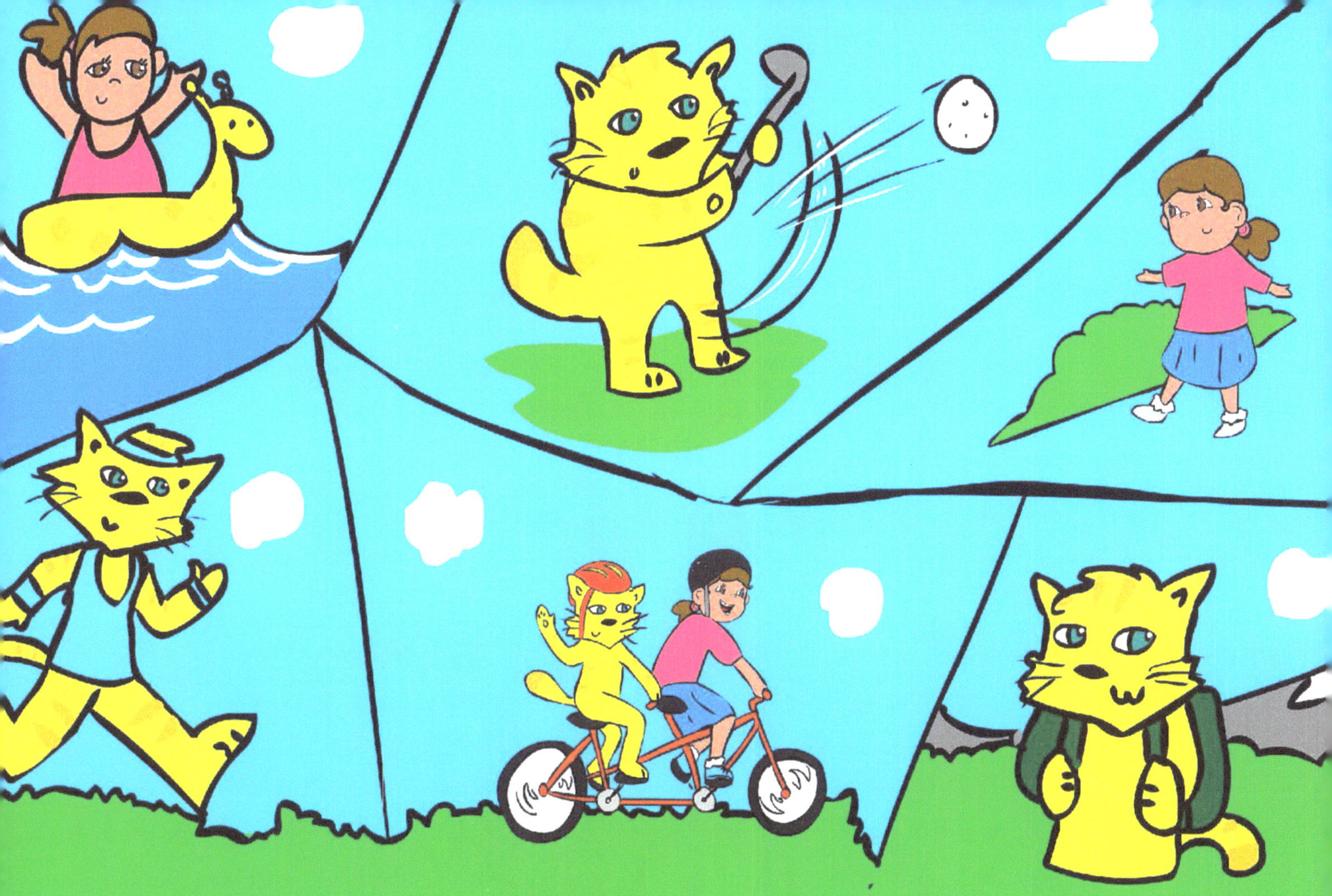

After eating there was nothing else for them to do.
But Layla had learned, that it just wasn't true.
"We could swim, we could golf, we could walk, we could run."
"We could bike, we could hike, we could do all sorts of fun."

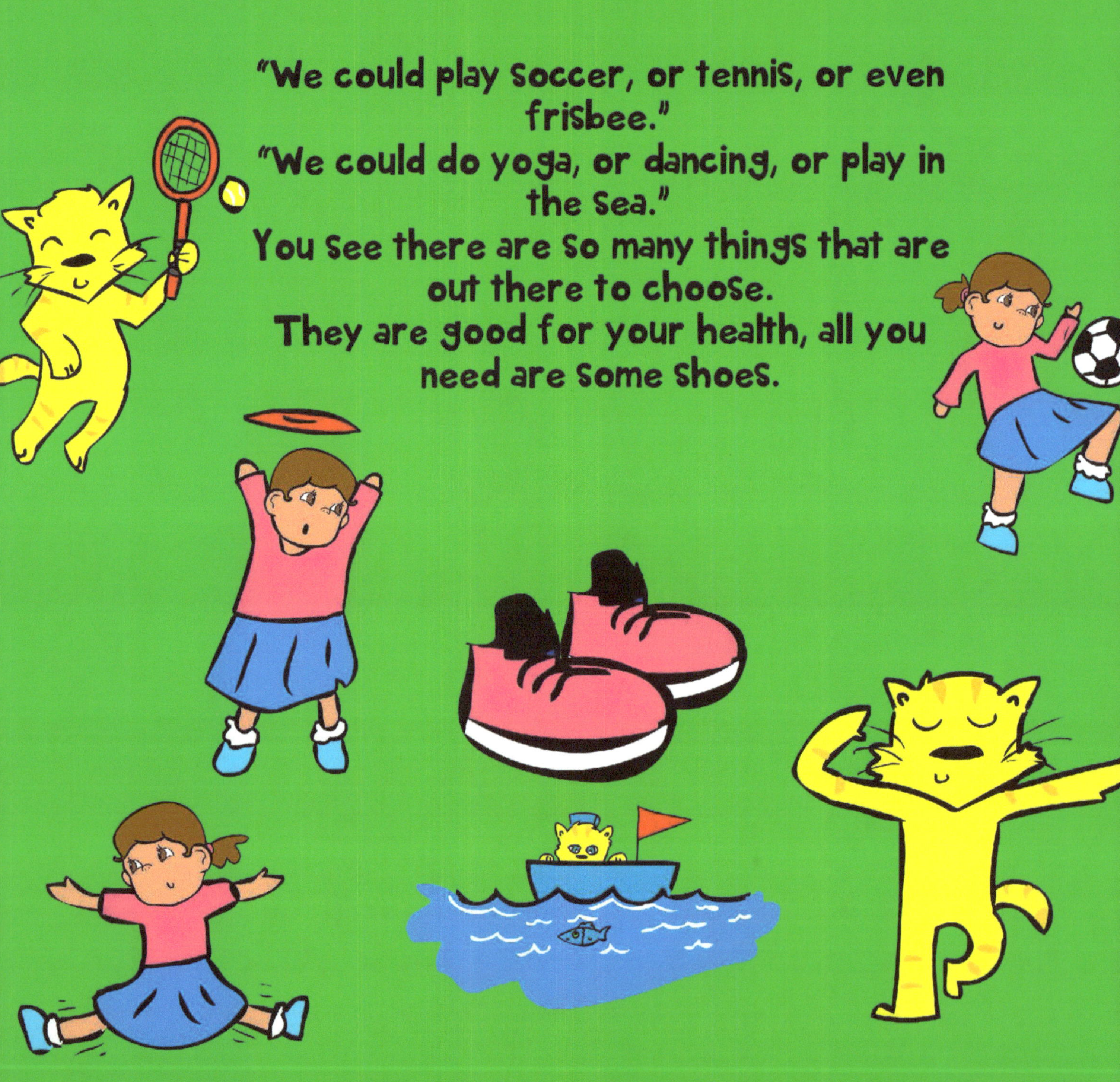

"We could play soccer, or tennis, or even frisbee."
"We could do yoga, or dancing, or play in the sea."
You see there are so many things that are out there to choose.
They are good for your health, all you need are some shoes.

To think that this morning Layla thought there was nothing
to do. Today she learnt that it just wasn't true.
Look at what happened, See it is not that strange.
She got out of bed, all it took was that change.

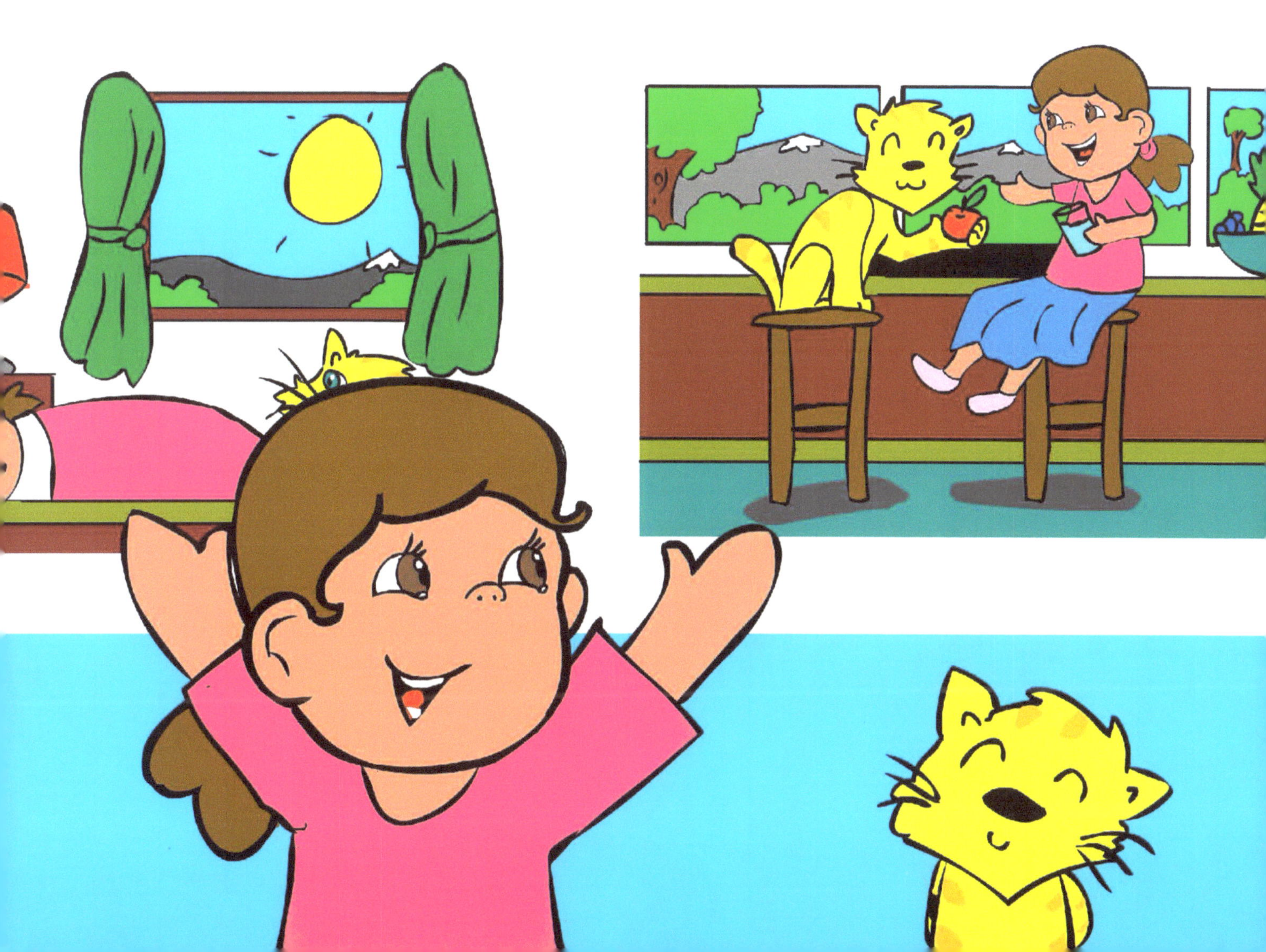

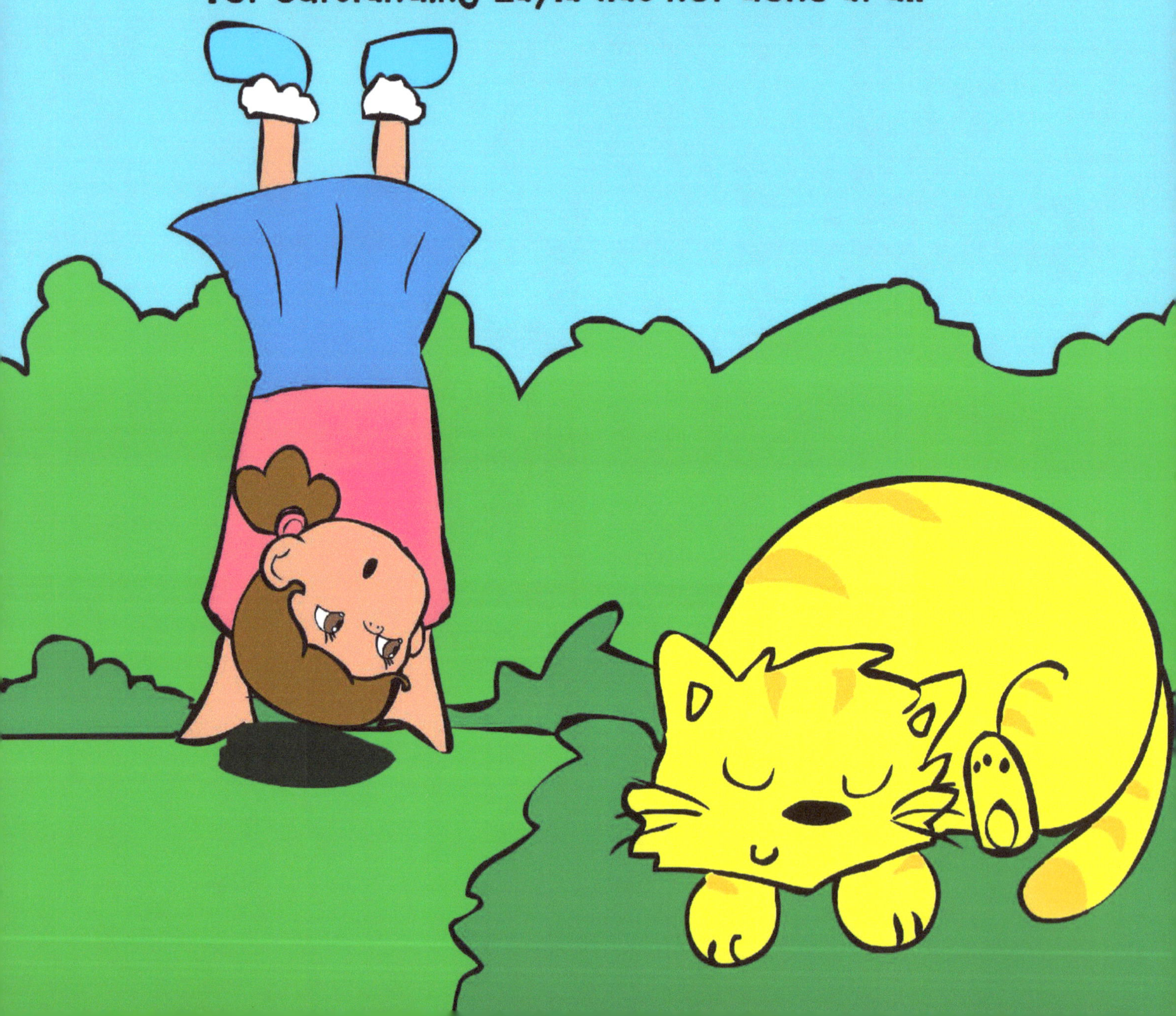
She took one step in the right direction
Layla and Ollie had a day of perfection.
Now Ollie was tired, and curled up in a ball.
Yet outstanding Layla was not done at all

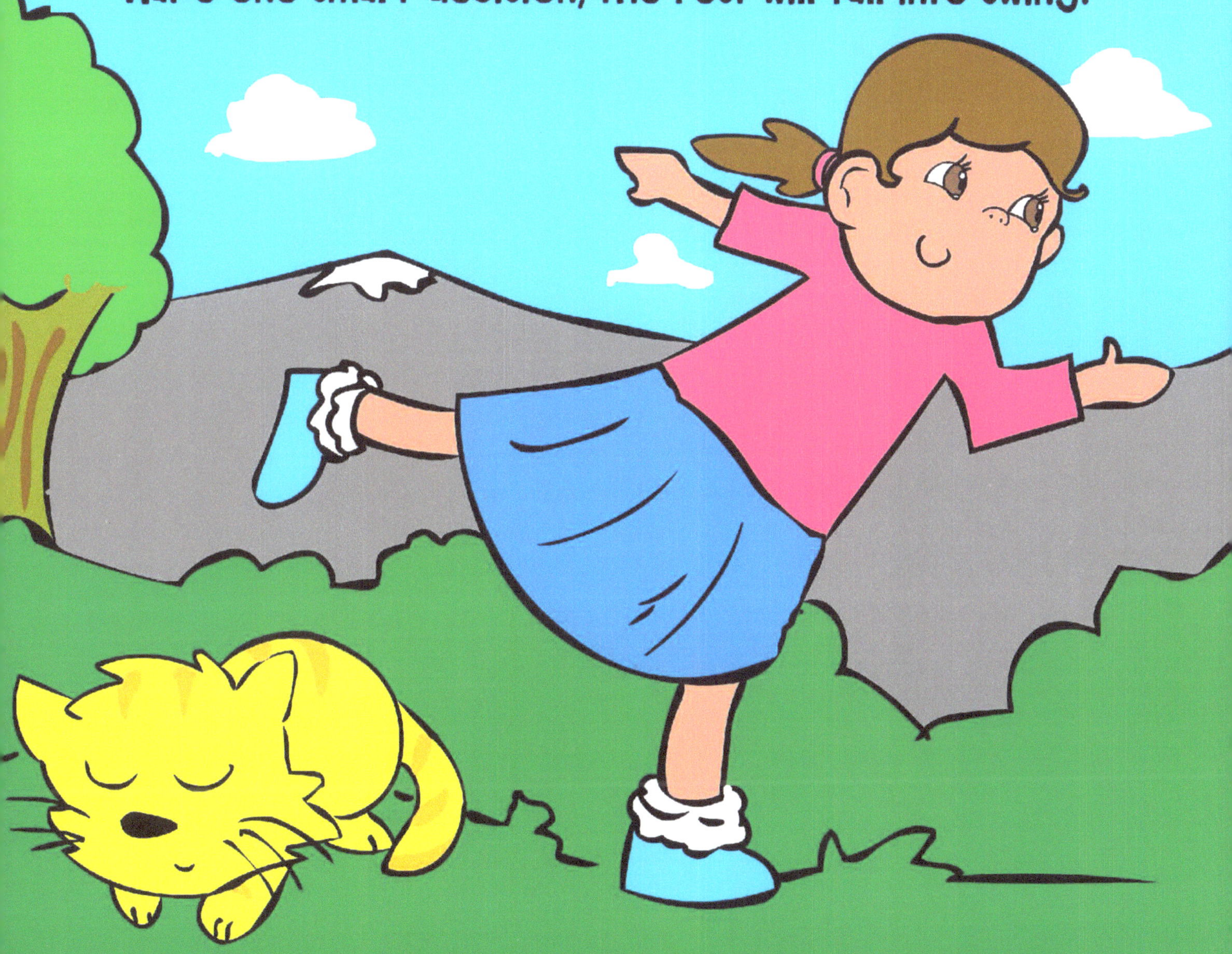

She started to practice her forward bend.
She couldn't wait for the morning to show her little friend.
She had a fantastic day by changing one thing.
Make one smart decision, the rest will fall into swing.

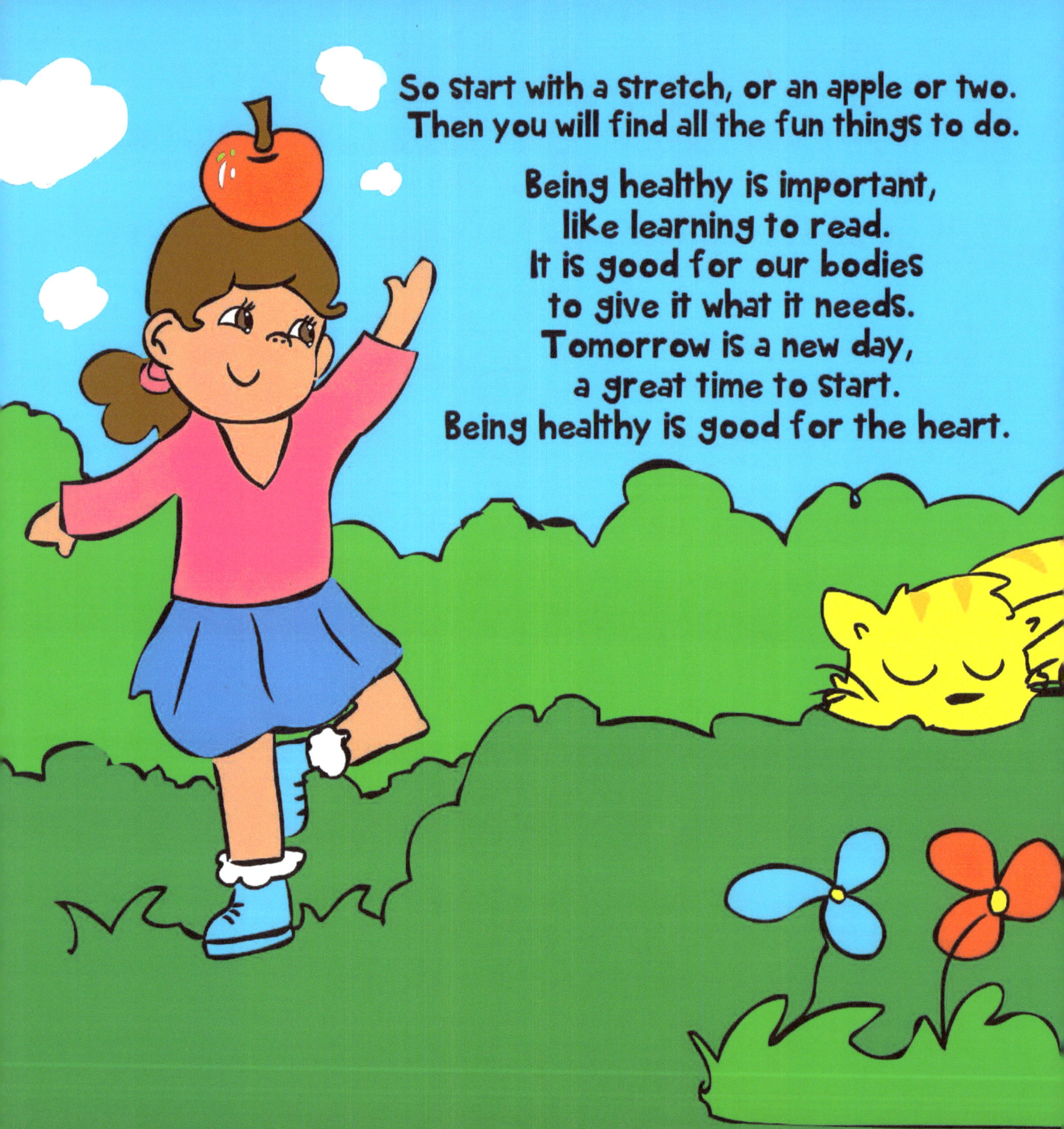

So start with a stretch, or an apple or two.
Then you will find all the fun things to do.

Being healthy is important,
like learning to read.
It is good for our bodies
to give it what it needs.
Tomorrow is a new day,
a great time to start.
Being healthy is good for the heart.

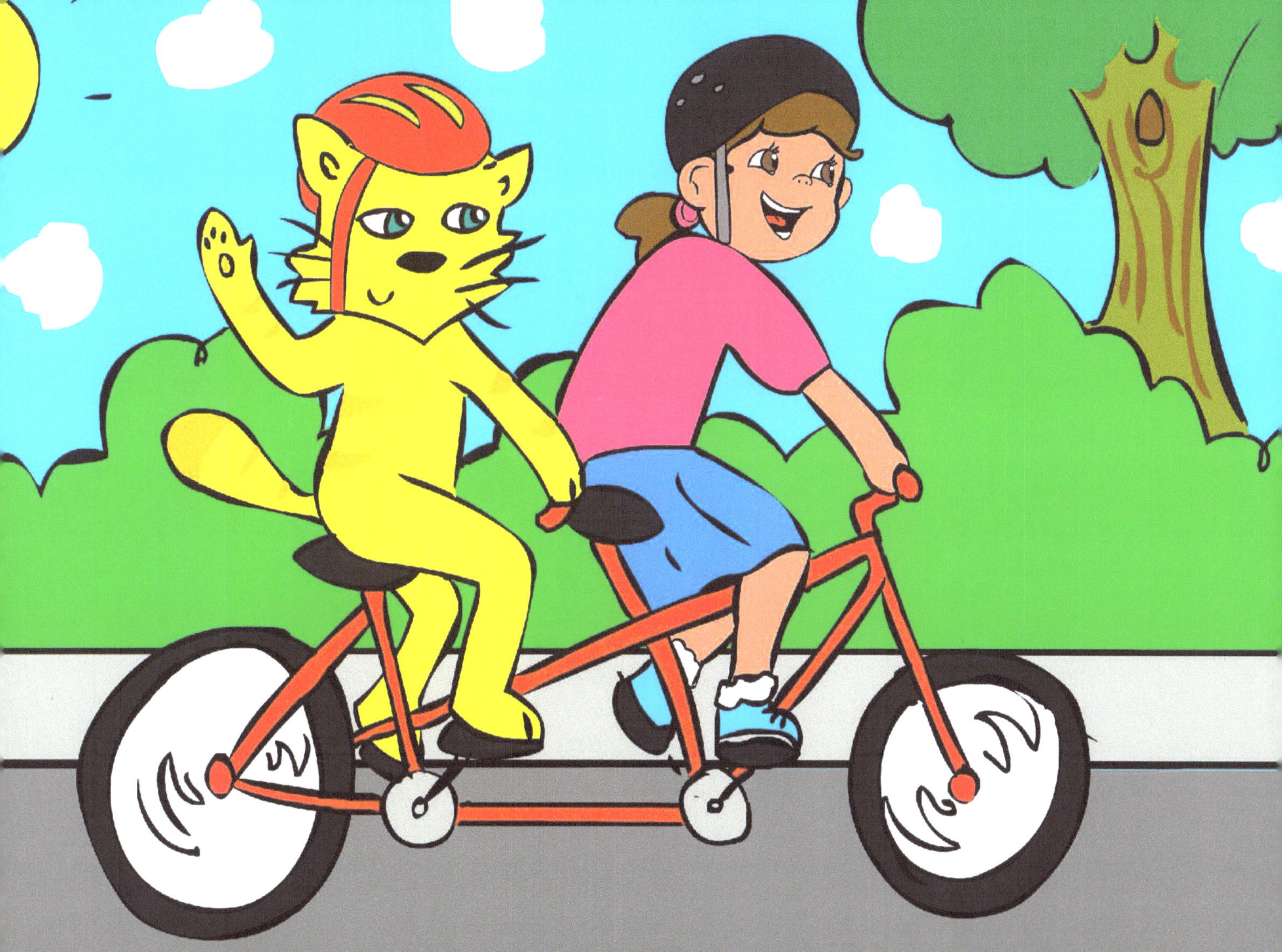

For Ollie and Layla, their fun has only just begun.
You might see them sometime when you go on a run.
Good luck and remember that whatever you do.
To try and make it healthy, and do what's best for you.

THE END

9 781976 553707